Qigong Flow
for Brain
Optimization

Improve Mental Clarity With

Qigong Daily Routine Exercises

Dan Phillips PhD

1

~DEDICATION~

~LARRY~

For your unwavering support, encouragement, and friendship. Your presence in my life has been a constant source of inspiration. Thank you for your invaluable kindness and belief in my journey. This book is a token of appreciation for your enduring friendship and steadfast encouragement.

TABLE OF CONTENT

CHAPTER 1: INTRODUCTION TO QIGONG AND
BRAIN OPTIMIZATION
- EXPLORING THE ANCIENT PRACTICE OF QIGONG
AND ITS MODERN APPLICATIONS FOR BRAIN
HEALTH
- THE CONNECTION BETWEEN MIND, BODY, AND
ENERGY IN QIGONG PHILOSOPHY
- SETTING THE STAGE FOR USING QIGONG TO
ENHANCE MENTAL CLARITY AND OPTIMIZE BRAIN
FUNCTION

CHAPTER 2: FOUNDATIONS OF QIGONG PRACTICE
- UNDERSTANDING THE KEY PRINCIPLES AND
CONCEPTS OF QIGONG PRACTICE
- BREATHING TECHNIQUES AND THEIR ROLE IN
IMPROVING OXYGENATION AND BRAIN FUNCTION
- THE IMPORTANCE OF PROPER POSTURE,
RELAXATION, AND ALIGNMENT FOR OPTIMAL
ENERGY FLOW

CHAPTER 1

Introduction to Qigong and Brain Optimization

It is now essential to pursue mental clarity and optimal brain function in our fast-paced environment of constant digital connectedness and information overload. This chapter delves into the ancient Chinese philosophy-based practice of Qigong and examines its remarkable relationship to brain health. We explore the harmonious relationship between the mind, body, and energy, laying the foundation for using Qigong to improve mental clarity and maximize brain function in the contemporary period.

Qigong's Age-Old Wisdom:

Pronounce it "chee-gong," qigong has its roots in ancient China and dates back thousands of years. Trained in Taoism, Confucianism, and Buddhism, Qigong arose as a comprehensive system that cultivated life force energy, called "Qi" or "Chi," for general health. It includes a broad variety of approaches, including as focused breathing exercises, meditation techniques, and mild postures and movements. Qigong is unique in that it emphasizes the connection between the mind, body, and energy inside the human system, using a holistic approach.

Contemporary Uses for Mental Health:

Even while Qigong was developed in an era far different from our own, its importance is still undoubtedly strong. The uses of Qigong in the present day go beyond its conventional intellectual and spiritual foundations. Numerous advantages that Qigong can provide for brain health and cognitive enhancement have been revealed by research. According to studies, regular Qigong practice may increase learning, mcmory, and mental agility by enhancing neuroplasticity, or the brain's ability to remodel and adapt.

The Link Between Mind, Body, and Energy:

The idea of connectivity is central to Qigong philosophy. It makes the argument that the body, mind, and energy are not separate entities but rather different aspects of one cohesive whole. The body's physical state is shaped by the mind, which also affects the flow of energy in this complex tapestry. This theory is in line with contemporary scientific understandings of psychosomatic interactions, which are processes in which mental moods affect physiological functions.

The mind, body, and energy link of Qigong is reflected in its practices. Mindfulness guides the movements, which are infused with intention and synced with breath. The motions themselves serve as channels that allow energy to freely circulate and nourish each and every cell and system. These components work together harmoniously to generate an atmosphere that supports brain improvement.

Contextualizing Brain Optimization:

It is important to understand that the road ahead does not lead to sudden enlightenment as we set out to utilize Qigong's ability for brain optimization. Instead, it's a process that calls for commitment, tolerance, and a willingness to learn about oneself. Qigong is a toolkit for gradually developing mental clarity and resilience rather than a magic wand that would instantly solve every cognitive issue.

The practical applications of Qigong—learning activities intended to increase mental clarity, stimulate brain activity, and support cognitive well-being—will be covered in the upcoming chapters. We will investigate the science underlying Qigong's effects on neurogenesis and neuroplasticity, providing insight into how these mechanisms support enhanced cognitive performance.

Through accounts from people who have witnessed Qigong's profound benefits on their cognitive capacities, we will acquire understanding of the potential and opportunities that lay ahead. The chapters will explore the various ways that Qigong interacts with brain health, extending beyond the physical to encompass spirituality and inner growth, from stress reduction to cmotional balance.

Qigong provides a haven in the fast-paced, stress-filled modern world whcn mental exhaustion and stress are widespread. It is a place where energy may flow freely, the body can regenerate, and the mind can find some peace. We will uncover the wisdom of old traditions and combine it with modern scientific understanding as we delve deeper into the practices and ideas of Qigong, setting the groundwork for a life of improved mental clarity and optimal brain function.

The next few chapters will move us from the theoretical to the practical side of things, with Qigong activities aimed at improving mental clarity taking center stage. We will work through the nuances of a daily Qigong routine designed for brain optimization, from an appreciation of the significance of good posture and breathing to the integration of mindfulness and visualization techniques.

Open your mind and heart to the adventure ahead, for the field of Qigong holds the key to reawakening the brain's latent energies, illuminating the paths leading to clarity, and directing your route toward a more energetic, concentrated, and optimal mental state.

CHAPTER 2

Foundations of Qigong Practice

- Understanding the key principles and concepts of Qigong practice
- Breathing techniques and their role in improving oxygenation and brain function
- The importance of proper posture, relaxation, and alignment for optimal energy flow

Qigong is a holistic technique that cultivates the body's vital force, also known as "Qi" or "Chi." It is an ancient Chinese practice with roots in traditional Chinese medicine and philosophy. In Chapter 2, the fundamental ideas and principles of Qigong practice are explored, with a focus on the practice's significant effects on mental, spiritual, and physical health. This chapter delves into the complex interactions between posture, energy alignment, breathing exercises, and relaxation, all of which support the improvement of Qi flow and general health.

Knowing the Essential Ideas and tenets of Qigong Practice:

A profound awareness of the human body as a dynamic energy system that is closely connected to the universe is at the core of Qigong. The basic ideas and concepts that form the basis of Qigong practice are introduced to practitioners in this chapter. One such idea is that Qi, which flows through the body's meridians or channels, is the essential energy that gives rise to all life. Health and well-being depend on the harmonious and balanced circulation of Qi, and Qigong is a potent technique for promoting this equilibrium.

The chapter also presents the idea of Yin and Yang, the dualistic forces that characterize the natural order of the universe. Achieving equilibrium between these complimentary and opposing energy is essential to Qigong practice. Practitioners can modify their activities to help themselves regain equilibrium by seeing Yang as the active, energizing force and Yin as the receptive, soothing energy.

Breathing Methods and How They Help with Brain Function and Oxygenation:

A key component of Qigong's effectiveness is the practice of mindful, deliberate breathing. The chapter's transformational effect of breathwork on brain function and oxygenation is highlighted in this section. Breathing slowly, deeply, and mindfully is a technique taught to Qigong practitioners. This improves oxygen intake and sets off the body's relaxation response.

Empirical studies have demonstrated that the intentional breathing methods used in Qigong practice activate the vagus nerve, which in turn facilitates relaxation, lowers stress levels, and enhances mental clarity overall. The brain's oxygen-rich blood flow optimizcs cognitivc proccsscs, resulting in enhanced emotional stability, attention, and concentration. Qigong breathing is rhythmic, which hclps practitioners become more attentive, rooted in the present, and developing a strong mind-body connection.

The significance of alignment, relaxation, and proper posture for optimal energy flow

This section of the chapter emphasizes how important alignment, relaxation, and good posture are to a successful Qigong practice. The body is thought of as a vessel for Qi, and the easy passage of this essential energy is greatly aided by the proper alignment of the body. Erroneous alignment can block energy channels, resulting in inertia and discord.

A variety of postures used in Qigong encourage alignment, flexibility, and relaxation. Through the adoption of these poses, practitioners facilitate the free flow of Qi, avoiding energy obstructions and promoting equilibrium both physically and energetically. The spine, which is sometimes called the "axis of Qi," is described in this chapter as having to be gently extended in order to facilitate Qi's free passage through the meridians.

Furthermore, emphasis is placed on relaxation as a mental and emotional state in addition to a physical one. Qi flow is thought to be disrupted by tension, worry, and anxiety; Qigong provides methods for letting go of these negative energies. By practicing mindful relaxation, practitioners can release tension and open up an area that is conducive to the development and flow of Qi.

Qigong is a holistic practice that treats the mind, spirit, and physical body as one whole. Crucial elements of the practice include bringing the mind into harmony with the body's motions and centering one's intention around the breath and flow of energy. This chapter helps practitioners become more focused and clear-headed so they can direct Qi to particular parts of the body for restorative and revitalizing effects.

To sum up:

In Chapter 2, the basic ideas and principles of Qigong practice are explored, along with the complex interrelationships between posture, energy alignment, breathing, and relaxation. The age-old wisdom of

Qigong is still relevant today as a potent way to improve mental clarity, bodily health, and spiritual well-being. Through the comprehension and acceptance of these fundamental components, practitioners set out on a metamorphic path towards balancing their Qi, promoting life, and developing a deep sense of overall equilibrium.

CHAPTER 3

The Brain-Body Connection
- Delving into the science behind the brain-body connection in Qigong practice
-    How   Qigong   impacts neuroplasticity, neurogenesis, and cognitive functions
- Exploring the role of Qi (energy) in influencing brain health and mental clarity

Qigong appears as a bridge in the complex dance between the mind and the body, bridging these two domains in ways science is only now beginning to comprehend. This chapter takes us on an intriguing journey into the realm of Qigong practice and the brain-body link. Explore the ways that Qigong affects neurogenesis, neuroplasticity, and cognitive processes as we explore the depths of neuroscience and traditional knowledge. We also embrace the role that Qi, or life force energy, plays in forming brain health and improving mental clarity.

The Mergence of Contemporary Science with Age-Old Wisdom:

The concepts of Qigong and our comprehension of the intricacy of the brain are quite similar. Using methods that have been confirmed by scientific research over time, ancient practitioners were able to intuitively recognize the connection between the mind and body. The comprehensive approach of Qigong is in perfect harmony with the understanding that the brain is an integral part of the body, interconnected with its physiological and energy systems.

The Adaptive Brain and Neuroplasticity:

The fundamental idea behind Qigong's impact on brain health is neuroplasticity, which refers to the brain's amazing capacity to change and reorganize its wiring in response to events. Qigong exercises activate brain networks and promote the creation of new synaptic connections because they place a strong emphasis on concentrated movements, breathing techniques, and awareness. This strategy builds resilience against age-related cognitive loss in addition to improving cognitive functions.

The Brain's Fountain of Youth: Neurogenesis

Interestingly, Qigong may also contribute to neurogenesis, which is the formation of new neurons in the hippocampus, an area of the brain important for memory and learning. Although it was long thought that this phenomenon was limited to the early stages of development, new study indicates that this ability is still present in the adult brain. By means of the complex fusion of Qigong's physical motions, breathing techniques, and mental concentration, practitioners can promote the growth of new neurons, thus enhancing cognitive vitality.

The Function of Qi in Mental Well-Being and Clarity:

A fundamental idea in Qigong philosophy is Qi, the unseen life force energy that permeates all living things. Regarding mental well-being, Qi is the medium via which essential energy nourishes and maintains mental processes. Stress, cognitive deterioration, and mental fog can result from blocked or imbalanced Qi. Qigong exercises aim to control Qi flow, allowing it to move freely and enhancing mental clarity and brain health as a result.

The Attuned Mind and Cognitive Boosts:

Qigong's focus on mindfulness, or being aware of the present moment, is essential for improving cognitive abilities. Research has demonstrated that practicing mindfulness can lower stress, sharpen attention, and enhance memory. Intentional breath control combined with the movements and postures of Qigong create a state of heightened awareness that nourishes the mind's ability to concentrate and focus.

Complete Health for a Developing Brain:

As the complex mechanisms by which Qigong affects the brain become clearer, the practice provides benefits beyond improved cognition. It addresses mental equilibrium, spiritual alignment, and physical wellness in a comprehensive manner. When these elements are balanced, an atmosphere is produced that supports brain optimization on several levels.

Traversing the Future Course:

Examining the relationship between the brain and body in Qigong practice reveals a tapestry made from the interwoven strands of contemporary science and traditional wisdom. It opens up a world of possibilities to realize that our thoughts, actions, and even the flow of Qi can influence our brains' fate. We take proactive measures to improve mental clarity, promote cognitive growth, and start a journey of self-discovery by incorporating Qigong into our life.

We will explore the real-world uses of this deep understanding in even more detail as we move through the upcoming chapters. Our trip will take us from particular Qigong exercises that target cognitive functions to a thorough grasp of how stress reduction affects the brain. Qigong has the power to reshape our mental landscapes. Accept this chapter as a link between conventional wisdom and contemporary research, working together to achieve the best possible mental clarity and brain health.

CHAPTER 4

**Qigong Exercises for Mental
Clarity**

**- Introducing a variety of Qigong
exercises specifically designed to
enhance mental clarity**

**- Step-by-step instructions for
practicing exercises that stimulate
brain activity**

**- Incorporating mindfulness and
visualization techniques to sharpen
focus and concentration**

With its deep connection to the mind and body, Qigong provides a wealth of exercises designed to improve mental clarity and acuity. This chapter explores a number of Qigong exercises that are carefully crafted to improve mental health and cognitive performance. These breathing, movement, and visualization exercises are designed to increase brain activity, improve focus, and cultivate a more profound feeling of mindfulness.

Presenting an Assortment of Qigong Exercises Particularly

Tailored to Promote Mental Clarity:

The holistic concept of Qigong acknowledges the connection between the mind and body. This chapter's exercises are carefully chosen to take advantage of this relationship and use it to improve mental clarity. These exercises provide a comprehensive strategy for preserving cognitive health by taking cues from centuries-old Qigong traditions and modernizing them.

An exercise that is highlighted is called "Five-Element Brain Activation." This practice, which has its roots in the Five Elements theory of traditional Chinese medicine, uses focused intention and gentle movements to stimulate the meridians corresponding to each element. Practitioners can foster a balanced flow of Qi throughout the body, supporting mental clarity and cognitive performance, by opening these energy conduits.

How to Practice Brain-Stimulating Exercises: A Step-by-Step Guide

This section gives practitioners step-by-step directions for conducting Qigong exercises that are specifically designed to increase activity in the brain in a simple and succinct manner. Every exercise is thoroughly described so that even those who are unfamiliar with Qigong can easily incorporate it into their regular regimen.

The "Crane's Wisdom Dance" exercise, for example, is included and involves flowing motions that mimic a crane's graceful dance. This exercise improves balance on a physical level while simultaneously stimulating neural connectivity and cognitive vibrancy by coordinating movements in both hemispheres of the brain. The exercise is broken down into digestible steps in this chapter, and practitioners are guided through concentrated intention, breath synchronization, and good posture.

Enhancing Concentration and Focus by Using Visualization and Mindfulness Techniques:

Exercises involving mindfulness and visualization are essential parts of Qigong for mental clarity. The focus of the chapter is on how practicing mindfulness, or being totally present in the moment, might improve cognitive function through increasing sensory awareness. Through the practice of mindfulness, individuals can enhance their cognitive processing and mental clarity by becoming acutely aware of the minute details in their body's movements and energy flow.

Additionally, visualization exercises are presented as effective means of improving concentration and focus. These practices entail visualizing energetic channels, balanced Qi flow, and alive energy inside the body.

During Qigong exercises, practitioners can concentrate focused imagery to improve the brain's ability to form new neural connections and strengthen existing ones. The exercises' cognitive effects are enhanced by the synergy between movement and imagination, which promotes mental resilience and clarity.

To sum up:

A series of Qigong activities that have been carefully selected to improve mental clarity and cognitive performance are revealed in Chapter 4. These Qigong-inspired workouts combine movement, breathing, mindfulness, and visualization techniques in a seamless way to promote brain health. By incorporating these techniques into their daily routine, practitioners can fully utilize the potential of their mind-body connection, leading to increased concentration, heightened focus, and a deep sense of cognitive vibrancy. With the lines between traditional knowledge and contemporary research becoming increasingly hazy, Qigong provides an ageless route to realizing the full capacity of the human mind.

Chapter 5: Daily Qigong Routine for Brain Optimization

- Designing an effective daily Qigong routine tailored to brain health

- A detailed guide to combining various exercises into a comprehensive practice

- Tips for integrating Qigong seamlessly into your daily schedule for maximum benefits

Being consistent is essential to achieving the best possible mental clarity and brain health. This chapter reveals the steps for a daily Qigong regimen created specifically to maximize the benefits of this age-old technique for brain improvement. Movement, breathing, and mindfulness are combined to produce a symphony that vibrates across our neural pathways, supporting mental health and cognitive processes. Prepare yourself for a daily metamorphosis in which every action becomes a brushstroke in the masterpiece that is your brain's vitality.

Creating a Daily Qigong Schedule:

Developing a daily practice of Qigong calls for intentionality and customization. Start by recognizing your bodily and cognitive demands at this moment. Are you looking for better concentration, less tension, or a calmer mind? Customize your regimen to meet your unique objectives. Remember that consistency is more important than intensity; it's best to begin slowly and build up the duration and intricacy of your practice over time.

The Elements of Qigong for Brain Optimization:

Your everyday practice of Qigong should be a harmonious fusion of breathing exercises, movement, and meditation. Start with light warm-up activities to arouse your body and get it ready for the workout. Include exercises that focus on cognitive processes, such as body-midline crossings that activate both hemispheres of the brain.

After you've completed the breathing exercises, move on to deep breathing exercises. Breathe in a rhythm that matches your actions to create a flow that energizes your body and soothes your mind. Lastly, wrap out your program with meditation exercises that promote introspection and inner peace. Taking a comprehensive strategy guarantees that you take care of the various facets of brain optimization.

A Thorough Practice Manual:

Divide your daily Qigong practice into small, reasonable chunks to make it accessible and efficient. Start with a quick warm-up to get your joints and muscles moving. Then proceed to the core of your program, emphasizing motions that encourage the flow of energy and activate cognitive processes. Include activities that test your equilibrium and motor skills, stimulating previously dormant brain regions.

Smoothly proceed from one exercise to the next, letting your breathing dictate the cadence of your routine. During every workout, practice mindfulness in your movements. Imagine the energy, or Qi, flowing through your body, feeding every cell and neuron. When you are in this elevated consciousness, you open up a channel for better brain function.

Application in Everyday Life:

A daily practice of Qigong is beautiful because it is so easily accessible. Take advantage of moments throughout the day to include Qigong into your everyday practice. Set the tone for the day ahead of yourself by practicing for a few minutes in the morning. Take short breaks from screens to practice a little Qigong to help clear your head. In the evening, embrace the relaxing effects of Qigong to decompress and get ready for a good night's sleep.

Keep in mind that consistency comes before duration. Doing mindful Qigong for even a little while each day might have a noticeable positive impact on your mental well-being. Maintain a journal to document your development and acknowledge minor successes, such as sharpened concentration, less anxiety, or an enhanced sense of general wellbeing.

Setting Out on a Transformative Journey:

You begin a life-changing adventure when you dedicate yourself to your daily Qigong practice; this journey takes place in the depths of your consciousness and reverberates through your physical tissues. Every action turns into a planned step toward improved mental acuity, cognitive performance, and general vitality. The beneficial changes you nurture through Qigong become ingrained in your neural architecture, producing a blueprint for long-term well-being, thanks to the plasticity of your brain.

We shall delve even further into particular exercises and practices that address emotional equilibrium and cognitive functions in the next chapters. You will see the significant influence that Qigong can have on your journey toward brain optimization as you include these practices into your everyday routine. Embrace this chapter as a compass that will lead you to a life of vivid mental clarity and wellness.

CHAPTER 6

**Stress Reduction and Cognitive
Enhancement**

**- Exploring the link between
chronic stress, cognitive function,
and brain optimization**

**- How Qigong's relaxation
techniques combat stress and
promote mental well-being**

**- Case studies highlighting
individuals who experienced**

cognitive improvements through stress reduction via Qigong

The harmful consequences of chronic stress on cognitive performance and general well-being have become more apparent in a world where demands are constant and life moves quickly. The complex relationship between stress, cognitive function, and Qigong's amazing ability to reduce stress and improve mental health is covered in detail in Chapter 6. The transforming impact of Qigong as a tool for stress reduction and cognitive enhancement is highlighted in this chapter through a thorough examination of relaxation techniques and engaging case stories.

Examining the Connection between Prolonged Stress, Mental Health, and Brain Enhancement:

Numerous studies have demonstrated the significant negative effects of long-term stress on cognitive performance. Repetitive activation of the stress response, which is the body's protective mechanism against danger, can make it maladaptive and have negative effects on the structure and function of the brain. Stress chemicals like cortisol can affect memory, focus, and judgment, which can ultimately impede cognitive function as a whole.

This chapter highlights the need of good stress management techniques by explaining the complex mechanisms via which long-term stress can cause cognitive deterioration. It also explores the idea of "allostatic load," which refers to the deterioration of the body and brain brought on by extended periods of stress. The accumulation of chronic stress might worsen cognitive impairment by causing oxidative damage and neuroinflammation.

How the Relaxation Techniques of Qigong Fight Stress and Advance Mental Health:

Its deep relaxation techniques are the foundation of Qigong's effectiveness in reducing stress. This chapter explores how Qigong's mind-body techniques mitigate the negative effects of stress and enhance mental health. The purposeful fusion of mindful breathing, slow, deliberate movements, and concentrated awareness in Qigong sets off the body's relaxation response, which in turn activates the parasympathetic nerve system and reduces the stress response.

Techniques like "Harmonizing Breath Meditation," which combines deep, slow breathing with imagery to create a profound level of calm, are taught to practitioners. In addition to lowering cortisol levels, this exercise improves heart rate variability, which is a crucial indicator of stress resilience. The chapter goes on to describe how the physical alignment and energy flow that are the focal points of Qigong help to reduce stress by clearing energy blockages and promoting stability and relaxation.

Case Studies Showcasing People Who Used Qigong to Reduce Stress

and Improve Their Cognitive Function:

Vivid case stories eloquently illustrate the transforming effects of Qigong in stress reduction and cognitive advancement. These true stories show people who started a Qigong journey to address long-term stress and saw significant improvements in their cognitive abilities.

In one case study, Sarah, a high-stress executive, is shown to be experiencing memory loss and mental exhaustion. By practicing Qigong regularly, Sarah was able to control her stress levels, which resulted in better decision-making, more mental clarity, and a revitalized feeling of energy. In a different case study, Alex, a student struggling with anxiety and academic expectations, is introduced. Alex was able to control his stress response thanks to Qigong's relaxing techniques, which also helped him focus better and succeed academically.

The aforementioned case studies demonstrate the beneficial effects of Qigong's all-encompassing stress reduction method on cognitive performance, highlighting the practice's capacity to lessen the long-term cognitive damage caused by stress and improve mental health in general.

To sum up:

In Chapter 6, the transformative potential of Qigong as a technique for stress reduction and cognitive enhancement is discussed, along with the crucial relationship between chronic stress and cognitive function. By thoroughly examining how stress affects the brain and the healing properties of Qigong's relaxation methods, practitioners get priceless knowledge on preserving and improving their mental well-being. Case studies from real life provide motivational evidence of Qigong's ability to reduce stress and build cognitive resilience. It also provides a way to improve one's well-being and cognitive vitality when faced with obstacles in life. As stress and cognitive function continue to collide in today's world, Qigong appears as an age-old cure for reestablishing equilibrium and mental optimization.

CHAPTER 7

Qigong and Emotional Balance

- Examining the relationship between emotional well-being and brain health
- Qigong exercises that target emotional centers in the brain to improve mood and stability
- Harnessing Qi to cultivate emotional intelligence and resilience

In the complex web of human experience, mental health is a vital thread that runs through our attitudes, deeds, and social interactions. This chapter explores in detail the mutually beneficial relationship between mental health and emotional balance, highlighting the transformational power of Qigong in this area. When combined with mental activities that focus on the brain's emotional centers, Qigong can serve as a compass to help us develop emotional intelligence, resilience, and better moods.

The Emotional Dance and Brain Health:

Emotions are not only fleeting feelings; they have a profound impact on our cognitive processes and the structure of our brains. The brain's health can be negatively impacted by long-term stress, worry, and unpleasant emotions, which can affect memory, decision-making, and general cognitive function. Positive emotions, on the other hand, have been connected to improved cognitive function and even increased neuroplasticity. Acknowledging this interdependence, we utilize Qigong as an instrument to balance our emotional terrain.

Emotional Resonance with Qigong Exercises:

With its focus on energy flow and attention, qigong has the unusual ability to affect emotional states. Exercises including Qigong stimulate and open neural pathways in parts of the brain related to emotional processing. Endorphins and other neurochemicals that improve mood and reduce stress can be released by certain motions that promote deep breathing and gentle motions.

Include activities that encourage you to concentrate on feelings such as joy, appreciation, and compassion. By means of purpose and imagination, these exercises activate brain regions that promote pleasant emotions, so establishing an atmosphere that supports emotional balance.

Using Qi to Develop Emotional Intelligence:

Beyond providing a momentary escape from unpleasant feelings, qigong offers a route to developing emotional intelligence. Self-awareness, empathy, and the capacity to successfully control and navigate one's own emotions are all included in the concept of emotional intelligence. Qigong cultivates these abilities through emphasizing self-awareness and attentive presence.

Through practicing Qigong, you develop a close awareness of your emotional landscape's oscillations. You make room to see and accept your feelings without passing judgment with every breath. Emotional intelligence is built on this process of self-awareness, which enables you to handle your feelings with grace and wisdom.

Sturdiness and Qi's Power:

In Qigong, resilience—the capacity to overcome hardship—finds a supportive friend. Qi cultivation allows us to access a reservoir of internal power and flexibility. Similar to how Qi moves freely through the body, Qigong creates an emotional flow that empowers you to face obstacles in life with poise and tenacity. The focus placed by Qigong on harmony and balance strikes a chord with us, providing a haven of stability even during emotional upheavals.

The Way Ahead:

Keep in mind that the path ahead is one of discovery and development as you immerse yourself in the realm of Qigong and emotional equilibrium. Feel the minute changes in energy and emotion as you embrace each practice with an open hcart. Emotions no longer serve as roadblocks when viewed through the lens of Qigong; instead, they serve as stepping stones towards incrcased resilience and a deeper sense of self.

We will continue to hone our comprehension and application of Qigong's effects on emotional health in the upcoming chapters. You will learn about the profound knowledge that Qigong gives to assist navigate the constantly shifting currents of our inner worlds through personal accounts of those who have found emotional peace in the practice and useful techniques designed for emotional balance. Accept this chapter as a starting point for your journey toward emotional freedom and the significant changes it may make to your general physical and mental state.

CHAPTER 8

**Beyond the Physical: Spiritual
Growth and Brain Optimization**

The physical, mental, and spiritual
aspects of life come together on the
Qigong practice path, providing a
significant chance for overall well-
being. Chapter 8 explores the
complex relationship between Qigong
and brain optimization, focusing on
the sometimes ignored but profoundly

transformational field of spiritual growth. This chapter explores the spiritual aspects of Qigong and presents inspiring tales of people whose spiritual Qigong practices led to profound changes in their thinking. It does this by exploring the integration of Qigong with mindfulness, meditation, and introspection.

Talking About the Spiritual Aspects of Qigong Practice and How They Affect Brain Optimization

The roots of Qigong can be found in ancient Chinese philosophy, which views Qi as a force that transcends the material world and enters the spiritual and mental spheres. This chapter explores the profound spiritual aspects of Qigong, looking at how the practices and concepts of the practice foster a higher level of awareness and connection. The complex relationship between spiritual development and brain optimization is explained, emphasizing how Qigong's all-encompassing method fosters mental, spiritual, and physical life.

The cultivation, balancing, and harmony of energy that is the focus of

Qigong is closely related to the activation of higher cognitive functions. Qi cultivation is a spiritual path that changes the practitioner's inner landscape in addition to being a physiological procedure. Neural networks become more optimized with spiritual growth, resulting in increased consciousness and improved cognitive performance.

Linking Inner Exploration, Mindfulness, and Meditation with Qigong:

Inner exploration, mindfulness, and meditation are harmoniously combined to form the foundation of

Qigong's spiritual elements. This chapter's section explores the mutually beneficial relationship between Qigong and these activities, explaining how they all work together to optimizc thc brain. In spiritual Qigong, mindfulness—a state attained through purposeful attention to the present moment—is a fundamental component. Through the practice of mindful breathing and movement, practitioners develop heightened sensory awareness and focused attention, which in turn promotes improved brain connectivity and cognitive clarity.

Another essential element is meditation, which explores the depths of consciousness and self-awareness. The chapter examines how the meditative elements of Qigong facilitate a transition from the cacophony of daily living to a place of inner peace. By utilizing the brain's plasticity, meditation practitioners can create new neural pathways and improve cognitive flexibility.

Telling the Narratives of People Who Have Undergone Deep Cognitive Transformations through Spiritual Qigong Practices:

Through moving accounts of people whose spiritual Qigong practices had a profoundly positive impact on their lives, the chapter is brought to life. These accounts demonstrate the amazing changes in cognition brought about by spiritual development in Qigong.

Michael is one such story, who, stressed out and troubled by constant stream of ideas, found comfort in the spiritual aspects of Qigong. He was able to transcend mental clutter, enjoy improved mental clarity, and develop a deep sense of oneness via consistent practice. Sofia is introduced in a different story, where her spiritual

Qigong journey led to a significant viewpoint shift. Sofia's cognitive frontiers broadened as she descended into her consciousness via Qigong meditation, which resulted in an increase in creativity and a better comprehension of her own mind.

To sum up:

Chapter 8 explores the profound field of spiritual development in Qigong and ties mindfulness, meditation, and introspection to the practice's effects on brain optimization. The physical and spiritual aspects of Qigong work together to create a powerful synergy that improves consciousness, strengthens the mind, and promotes spiritual health. This chapter highlights how Qigong can help achieve transcendent cognitive transformations through the lens of personal talcs, cncouraging practitioners to go on a journey that is holistic and encompasses not just the physical body but also the mind and soul. In light of the convergence of spiritual development and brain optimization, Qigong becomes a key to releasing the latent potential of human consciousness and intellect.